GREG:
A Liver Transplant Recipient

GREGORY GAINES JR.

Bloomington, IN 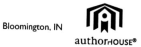 Milton Keynes, UK

authorHOUSE®

AuthorHouse™
1663 Liberty Drive, Suite 200
Bloomington, IN 47403
www.authorhouse.com
Phone: 1-800-839-8640

AuthorHouse™ *UK Ltd.*
500 Avebury Boulevard
Central Milton Keynes, MK9 2BE
www.authorhouse.co.uk
Phone: 08001974150

This book is a work of non-fiction. Unless otherwise noted, the author and the publisher make no explicit guarantees as to the accuracy of the information contained in this book and in some cases, names of people and places have been altered to protect their privacy.

First published by AuthorHouse 1/17/2007

ISBN: 978-1-4259-6906-6 (sc)

Printed in the United States of America
Bloomington, Indiana

This book is printed on acid-free paper.

CONTENTS

Acknowledgements

First of all, I want to take this time out to say thank you to Greg Sr, and Cynthia Gaines(my parents). Dad, thank you for being the role model that I've always needed. There are too many people who have never known what it's like to have a father like you because they've had to grow up without their father's love and guidance. I want to personally thank you for all the unsaid things that a son usually doesn't acknowlegde. Thank you for keeping clothes on our backs, keeping the electricity on and maintaining a roof over our heads. Most of all, thank you for equipping me with the life-lessons that have molded and sculpted me into the young man that I am. Mom, thank you for showing me a softer side of love and humility. It's because of you that I have a sensitive side and I'm not ashamed to admit it. The both of you have stood by each other and you've stood by me even when I really didin't deserve it. You've shown me what to do and what not to do in my life in my relationships. Those concepts are priceless to me. To Brian and Marcus (my younger brothers), thank you both for playing such vital roles in being part of my support system. Even if I have to use my own past mistakes as example references. I would also like to thank everybody in our extended family: The Gaines', The Millers, The Baxters, The Brockingtons and anybody else's name who slips my mind at the present time. I love you all. To my daughter Jamie, never again will I struggle to provide for you. From now on, daddy will make a way for you to live your life comfortably. As your father, I am not going to let you down in any way. I will always have your back. To my daughter's mother, thank you for believing in my writing. You told me that I had talent even before I started to realize it. Thank you for helping me to grow and being my friend and "partner in crime". Thank you to everybody at Boomtown dinner theatre and everywhere else that holds "open mic nights" for people like myself to display what's on their mind. Thank you to the medical staff at St.

Luke's Hospital and the Mayo Clinic for showing me love and concern for my well-being. Keep touching people's lives one patient at a time. Last but not least, I want to thank Mr. Greg Swaringen for being my true best friend for all these years. We've known each other since Elementary School, Greg, and I just want to say that I love you like a brother and I miss you. Thank you for just being you and relating to me on so many issues.

Introduction

To all who still to this day, believe that there is no God, I'm living proof that he <u>does</u> exist. Amid all of the medical trouble that I've been through, God's been with me the whole time. It's important for everyone to know that God is God. You can not manipulate, mitigate or berate God. We as human-beings sometimes get angry and blame God for all of our troubles. Murder, disease and suffering are not caused by God but he is always the first one we point our fingers at when these things happen. Understand this: If God acted more like a genie or Santa Clause, we would never change. Ever! We would never want to do anything for ourselves. We would all grow up physically but psychologically we wouldn't mature. Sometimes it takes a tragedy for us to see life clearly.

For other people it might have to take several tragedies for people to learn to take life more seriously. God is the way he is because whether we like it or not, we need sovereignty. If you think that God has never done anything for you, you're wrong. You could've been dead but instead you're still alive and you're listening to my words. It's vital for us to count our blessings and notice the little things in life. This is something that my writing has helped me to realize since I first started. Even though my writing isn't always "Christian oriented", it still gave me the opportunity to listen to myself. It helped me to be less demanding and more empathetic. Since I was a pre-teen, I've had to seek counsel from at least three shrinks but never once managed to make a breakthrough until I started writing two years ago. So writing is more than just fascinating to me, it's therapeutic. I'm not perfect though, I still make mistakes, sometimes repeatedly. I hope reading my story helps you to not only understand my struggles and my passions but other people's stories who are currently going through some of the same things. There are people who have gone through worse situations than mine and they're even younger than I am. For all transplant patients and recipients everywhere: This is my story, this is what happened........

CHAPTER 1
Who I Am

My name is Gregory Lloyd Gaines Jr. I was born on August 11, 1979 in Ft. Pierce, Florida. I'm the eldest of three kids bore from Gregory Sr. and Cynthia Gaines. My parents originally had four children with all of us being boys. Their second child, Adrian, is now deceased so I currently only have two younger brothers.

Ever since I was a little boy old enough to talk, I've always been a little carefree but I've had to spend most of my life in and out of hospitals. I was diagnosed with cirrhosis of the liver after my first two weeks of birth, due to biliary atresia, that turned my skin and eyes dark. Since having my first liver transplant at six years of age, I've been blessed enough to survive four more major surgeries throughout the twenty-seven years I've been alive. Growing up, I was very introverted and scared to share my thoughts and opinions with anyone.

I can remember that one of the very first feelings that I learned that stuck with me for the majority of my life was "shame". I used to have vivid flashbacks of back when I was in Elementary School. Anytime I made a failing grade or half completed an assignment, I was both confronted and criticized. It didn't just start or end in the classrooms either.

I've lived most of my life in fear and resentment, I was basically scared of my own shadow. It taught me to be extremely shy and anti-social. I also went through episodes of being humiliated and ridicule from my peers but kids are really cruel to each other when they don't know any better. School academics never were easy for me to handle.

I didn't know this at the time but I struggled all through school because I never really learned how to study properly. There were certain lessons and concepts in which I did catch on to but there were many that I could not grasp right off the bat. At first, I thought that studying was just simple memorization of class material including lessons, discussions and further reading material. Even when I hear myself spout off a generalized synopsis of what studying really is, it sounds incredibly self-explanatory and understandable. Well, as a matter of fact, it was so easy for me to comprehend that I failed at least 60% of all the written tests I had to take.

I can honestly admit with <u>no</u> shame that I thought I was stupid. I couldn't get over the fact that studying for tests came so easily to all my other classmates. Some of the teachers I had would always talk a good game and tried their hardest to convince me that they were there for me. Anytime I had to ask them a question about my assignments, they would make it seem like all I had to do was ask them but whenever I <u>did</u> ask them questions half of them became intolerant and just plain rude with me because of my finite understanding. I felt as if I had a learning disability and so I went about my studies as if I didn't care.

When it came time for all of the students to be dismissed from class for the day, I would stop at nothing to attempt to hide my failing grades and prevent my parents from finding out. By the time I got home from school, I found myself frantically scrambling around in my room shoving my assignments in any kind of unsuspecting crevice I could find.

Everytime my dad asked to see my folders, I would try to alleviate them of any blemished assignments and I would only show him my folders that had the good grades in them. Knowing I was dead wrong, I would always try to fabricate a story and explain as to what happened to the rest of my assignments to my father. The majority of the time, my father knew I was lying to him but being severely confronted about it on several occasions just wasn't enough for me to come clean and stop the lying. Of course the proof was always in the pudding though when it came time for report cards to come home.It was a very viscious cycle that I had created for myself: refuse to study for tests, half complete assignments and lie about the progress I <u>wasn't</u> making in school. I knew I could do better but didn't know how to go about making it happen for myself.

My problems were habitual and eventually got so bad for me that I was overcome with depression. I started having suicidal thoughts and writing suicidal notes to myself. I didn't know what else to do, I felt like a failure most of the time. Around the time I was 14 or 15, I was psychologically evaluated and diagnosed with having A.D.D. or attention deficit disorder and was prescribed the medication ritalin to help me concentrate. I finally had a medical term that explained at least some of the problems I battled while I was in school. The other 50% of my problems were purely intentional on my part.

CHAPTER 2
My Medical Obstacles

I'm sure that you understand what I went through in school now but I struggled with life both inside and outside of the classrooms. I've had to adapt to <u>not</u> living a normal life three times since I was 6 years old because of my transplants. I was born with a brown-skinned complexion before my jaundice got the best of my body's immunity.

When I became jaundiced, my eyes and urine turned dark yellow. My skin also turned very dark and my blood became infected with toxins that made me itch all the time. These symptoms will render you fatigued and a little irritable. Before my first transplant, I had never experienced the "never-ending" energy and zest for life that usually normal kids experience because I was always scratching. It's almost like having the "chicken-pox" except there are no bumps so you scratch constantly.

Chicken-pox usually goes away after a couple to a few weeks depending on how strong your immune system is, yellow jaundice from liver failure stays in your body for a lot longer. Doctors have since dramaticlly improved combating organ rejection with certain immuno-suppressive prescription medications but it used to be that things wouldn't get any better for you until you've been placed on a waiting list to receive a new liver.

They first have to determine your blood type and categorize you medical urgency. The severity of your medical predicament determines where you're placed on the list. If your situation isn't that severe, don't hold your breathe on hoping you receive your transplant exactly when <u>you</u> want it, there's a process that has to take place. The donor of a liver has to die first and then your blood type has to match the donor's, otherwise, the organ will be completely incompatible with your body's immunity regardless of what medications you take.

Then depending on your medical situation and how emergent it is, the Board of Trustees has to debate and vote on who gets the donated organ and why. When the organ becomes available, that's when transplants are granted. They're very pricey surgeries though, they cost on average between $250 to $300,000. There are literally thousands of people waiting for livers every year so you're going to have to take it one day at a time until your number is up for you to be transplanted.

Meanwhile, my thinking had to be re-conditioned for me to continue to survive and thrive. The hardest thing for me to accept was that I was not a normal kid and never will be.

On January 17, 1985, my first born younger brother, Adrian, was conceived. He was a sick baby as well as myself. He was diagnosed at birth with having congenital heart disease and was also frequently hospitalized. It saddens me to say that I don't really remember much about him because he was born right before I received my first transplant. I have pockets of slight memories from when I used to try to entertain him but I was only 5 years old at the time. Now that I really reminisce, I do remember a few scenarios of when he was coughing severely.

Adrian live for two months after his birth when he abruptly caught a bad case of pneumonia and died in March of 1985. I remember seeing him in the hospital once he was hooked up to all kinds of tubes before his death. At that precise second, I did not recognize him at all, I honestly thought he was someone else. At his funeral, I did feel somewhat sad but I was too young to experience real grief.

The gravity of losing my brother didn't hit me until much later in life. My parents were devastated though. <u>Nobody</u> should ever have to bury their own child, it should be the other way around. Doctors tending to Adrian before his death told my parents that he would need at least three more open heart surgeries throughout his life if he was going to continue to survive. After his death, my parents then made the difficult decision to donate his organs so that he could live on in someone else's child. He would've been an adult by now, he's only six years younger than I am. I wonder how he would've turned out.

On one summer night in 1986, my liver failure became critical. I fell into a coma with a very serious nose bleed and had to be air-lifted to the Children's Hospital in Pittsburg, Pennsylvania. I received my first liver transplant on July 10, 1986. I was the 300th some odd patient who was operated on by Dr. Thomas Starzle. Dr. Starzle was the man who pioneered organ transplantation and so wherever he was, there stood my best chance for survival at the time. Back then in the early 1980s, transplantation was still experimental, it hadn't graduated to a normal surgery yet. When all the madness ended, I was placed on <u>several</u> immuno-suppressive medications that had mild side effects but for the most part, things were looking up for me and my family.

One of my medications called cyclosporin caused me to grow facial hair because of the large dosage I was prescribed. I had a full blown mustache at six and a half years of age. Another side effect was gingivitis from which called for me to have extensive gum reduction surgery. Later on in life, I would have other dental work done on my mouth.

I was also prescribed a steroid called prednisone, that stunted my growth which is why instead of standing at at least 5'10 tall, I'm only 5'6 ½. It makes your body retain water and it'll eventually render your bones brittle if taken in large dosages for a prolonged period of time. My mother had to stay in the Ronald McDonald House while also periodically staying overnight with me in the Children's House during my rehabilitation.

I remember making a few friends while I was there and one of them was a girl named Teresa. She became my very first girlfriend and for a short period of time, we were inseperable. There was just puppy love between us but we were two peas in a pod and we were seen everywhere together, even on the playgrounds and parkbenches. My mother knew her mother and we conversed with each other and had fun.

Despite the rough times of feeling like she was standing on pins and needles from having to watch her son fight for his life, my mother still had hope for me in her heart. She carried a smile on her face everywhere she went and she was easily befriended by anyone. My father was along with us for a small portion of my ordeal but he was trying to juggle both his job and making time to come see us.

It put a huge burden on both of my parents for having to sit through the anitcipation of my surgery but as much as my father wanted to be by our side, he also had to make sure he could continue to financially provide for us.

After at least three months of rehabilitation from my surgery, we finally said our goodbyes and thank-yous to the entire medical team and to all of the other parents whose children also received transplants. We made a move from Ft. Pierce, Florida to Orange Park, Jacksonville, Florida right before I recuperated.

CHAPTER 3
My Self-Esteem

When we got back home in Jacksonville, we were welcomed with a surprise block party that our neighbors threw for us. It was a "Welcome Back" type shindig but it was that very heartwarming gesture that made coming back all the sweeter.

Time progressed sooner than later and before I knew it, I started to smile and laugh out loud very often. I also started skipping and running, this might not be considered a big deal to a normal child but it wasn't normal to me because I had been fatigued and under other symptoms from my jaundice for so long that I didn't recognize myself. This was amazing, I felt like I had super powers (at least when I was that young that was how I felt) or something.

Life at this point seemed so much brighter to me. I stayed outside all day long playing without scratching. My skin cleared up and returned to the "medium brown" skinned complexion I was born with and I had developed little rock calf muscles from running so much. Thus from whence came my nickname "Rock" that was given to me by my grandfather. Little did I know the magnitude of that name. I was only a kid when it was given to me but I had no idea how powerful and how suitable it really was.

The first two and a half years after my transplant went by like a blur. I can honestly say that I don't think I ever had any bad days. Even if I did, I couldn't remember them because I was having too much fun to really care. I was completely oblivious to life's troubles and issues up until I was nine years old.

At the exact age of 9 was when I suddenly started to worry about my self-esteem. I also started viewing girls differently (attractively), they no longer had the "cooties" to me anymore. I started questioning my looks and I found myself checking my appearance out in the mirror on a consistent basis. I found quite a few females to be very pretty but unfortunately some of the same girls I felt so strongly for didn't feel the same way about me.

It started to really break my heart when girls wouldn't reciprocate their feelings back to me. I did what I could to show them that I was interested but most of my efforts were in vain. The low self-esteem I had from a lack of social skills hindered my communication skills so much that before I even tried to introduce myself to a girl, I would write her a love letter.

Now, normally this would be one of the most sincere forms of flattery (when you're young) and there wouldn't be anything wrong with it if the girl actually knew I existed first. I was just handing out love notes at random, hoping and praying that somebody would pay attention to me. Most times, right after a girl received one of my notes and read it, she would arrogantly look at me and laugh as if she was taking me for a joke. See, I've never been the type of guy to just attract females from afar. I've always had to try talking to them first.

My epiphany about females didn't come to me until much later in my life but what I didn't realize was that it wasn't that they thought I was unattractive. It was the fact that I was going about approaching them all in the wrong ways. Constant rejection will teach you to do some things differently. It would eventually take me twelve more years for me to learn to change my approach and that I <u>do</u> have something to offer a female in a relationship but it would be a long time coming.

Aside from having trouble talking to girls, I also perpetually had my work cut out for me with my studies. As I have said before, may lack of study skills continued to kill off any small amount of academic confidence I had left. By the grace of God, I got through Elementary School and High School by the skin of my teeth. With some prayer and a whole lot of hard work, I attained the necessary extra credits to graduate with my correct class: c/o '98.

I had to repeat the 8th grade because I was too occupied with being the class clown. My clown antics held me back a grade so it was highly important to me that I get back to where I needed to be academically.

CHAPTER 4
Medical Hope

After I graduated from High School, I became jaundiced from my liver again at the age of eighteen. The cause of my liver failure this time was due to me being immature with the handling of my suppressive medication. My family and I were down south in Fort Pierce, Florida visiting my grandparents. My parents had taken a cruise to Jamaica and had just came back to take my younger brothers (Brian and Marcus) and myself back home, when my mother noticed my eyes turning yellow again. Their hearts immediately dropped because their son was going to have to revisit being re-transplanted.

Luckily, they just started to become familiar with St. Luke's Hospital which is affiliated with the very reputable Mayo Clinic, here in Jacksonville, Florida.

When we sought their help, they were very clear and thorough with their procedures through their consultations. Once I was back on the waiting list for another liver, I waited patiently for the qualification process to progress for at least one year.

While I was anticipating my next transplant, my jaundice brought on a whole new set of problems. I had the usual itching sensation, darkened skin, the yellow eyes along with the fatigue and irritability but I had also developed cataracts from which took me having to get involved in three car accidents before I noticed how bad they had gotten. I didn't know what cataracts were at first. They got so bad that a glaucoma atttack occurred. I was 19 when I received cataract removal surgery prior to my last transplants.

The glaucoma damaged my right eye so much that my opthamologist said that it wouldn't have done any good to put another replacement lens there so he decided not to put one in. It's all right with me though. As long as I still have vision in one of my eyes, I'm fine. I will always be half blind for the rest of my life but I have come to terms with it among other things.

On the day of my second transplant, my surgeons discovered that this liver wasn't working the way it should've been. This made an unsatisfactory impression on my surgeons so much that they re-transplanted me with a third liver twelve hours later. The dates were December 31, 1999 and January 1, 2000 for my last liver so I received two livers back to back.

While I was patched up with stitches and bandages and still recuperating in my hospital room two days later, physical therapists came in my room to help make me move around. It wasn't like I fell down and sprained my ankle, I got cut <u>deeply</u>. I swear to God I wanted to choke the hell out of those physical therapists (sarcasm).

I eventually recuperated after a few months but the process went a little slower for me this time. By this time I'm 20 so I'm not the same bubbly little kid I once was at 6 when I was full of energy. Rehabilitating from all of the pain took a little longer to subside but I still made a remarkable recovery.

CHAPTER 5
Hard-Knock Life

Shortly after my 21st birthday, I met my daughter's mother via the internet. She was my very first serious girlfriend and our relationship progressed very quickly from our meet and greet interaction. After only being boyfriend and girlfriend for a little over a year, we moved in with each other. Morally, we knew we were wrong for shacking up without first getting married but we just wanted to escape the extra responsibilities that our parents were trying to enforce upon us.

We felt like they were just trying to antagonize us so therefore we had to break out in a mad dash to establish ourselves.

We were young and dumb but we thought that we were in love and from that point on <u>nobody</u> was going to tell us anything different. The both of us went through several roller coaster rides of emotions together because not only did we continue to rebel against our parents' advice and guidance but we fought each other. There were times when we <u>were</u> happy together but those days never lasted that long before we found something else to fight about.

One year since our move-in together, I surprisingly impregnated her with our baby girl. During the pregnancy we got along beautifully but no relationship is perfect, every one of them has their ups and downs. Ours overall was a bit more turbulent than others were. The one necessity we hardly ever had enough of was money. It was always either one of us was working or both of us were unemployed. We went days to weeks at a time where we had absolutely no money and no food. Our lights were cut off, our phone service was constantly getting disconnected and we were evicted from our first apartment complex.

The next apartment we went to was slightly more affordable but our struggle didn't exactly end there either. My father stopped by to visit on several occasions and tried to talk some sense into me about changing my situations but I was too head strong and ignorant to hear what he had to say. To attempt to make surviving easier for us to handle, my daughter's mother went to live with <u>her</u> mother in Tallahassee, FL so she could also go to school. On the morning of March 14, 2003 our little girl, Jamie, was born.

She was born 5lb. and 13oz., 19 inches long and had to be delivered by Cesarean section because her mother developed toxemia before giving birth to her. She's had to battle diabetes since she was younger so the doctors had to induce labor eight weeks short of the nine month period. Fortunately, I already had a new job by the time Jamie, arrived so after a couple of months both my daughter and her mother came back to Jacksonville, FL to live with me.

We tried to remain together and be the happy family that we should've been but it was no use. In late May of 2004, we had hit rock bottom and we were evicted for the last time from our second apartment. Whatever further obstacles that were headed our way, we were still going to handle them ourselves. We were pig-headed to the very bitter end and persistently refused to swallow our pride and seek refuge to our parents. We just couldn't find it within ourselves to retreat from poverty and seek a safe haven.

As a result, we lived in our cars for two weeks. We even sunk so low that we tried to live in the downtown shelters. As ridiculous as this sounds, I had a family of my own out on the streets, <u>homeless</u>. My daughter's mother managed to contact one of her college classmates from college and asked her if we could stay with her until were able to get back on our feet. Miraculously, her friend accepted and we stayed with her for one week.

While we were staying there, somehow word got around on the street that we had fell on really hard times and my father found out. I had previously assumed from all of the <u>disrespect</u> I showed him just before I hastily moved away that he was going to chastise me but actually he did the complete opposite. He wasn't exactly ecstatic to see me again especially on these terms but he still welcomed us with open arms and invited us to come back home until we got our ducks back in a row. He then decided to contact my daughter's mother's father so that she could have a safe place to dwell under as well. Right before our "coming back to the nest" plan became official I lost the previous job that I had.

Things kind of happened one after the other as in a domino effect. While life continued to beat us down, we finally had had enough of each other and decided to call our relationship off. We knew we were better off going our own separate ways, the relationship just wasn't working out anymore. Our break-up was even more bitter than our turbulent times together. We fought each other like cats and dogs and took turns stabbing each other in the back, calling out each other's name and so forth.

Since then, we have stopped fighting and have made amends. Instead of being die-hard enemies, we're friends now. I try to help her out as much as I can with our baby even if she needs a small break just to get some much needed rest. If and whenever she needs more financial assistance in regards to our little girl, if I can afford it, I gladly offer my help. We interact much better now than we ever did when we were together.

CHAPTER 6
The Transition Process

Some months had passed up to a year and then I ran into more medical trouble in late May of 2005. I had just got a new job and was currently working while I was under a mild fever when out of the blue, I felt as if I were about to pass out. My nose started to bleed and my fever worsened to the point of chills. My supervisor eventually sat me down, called an ambulance and I was immediately rushed back to St. Luke's Hospital. The first thing doctors did when I got to the hospital was try to sustain me with I.V. fluids and then several blood cultures were drawn. A spinal tap was conducted to test for various types of infections and the possibility of meningitis but those results came back negative.

By the way, I have a new-found respect for what pregnant women go through when they receive an epidural injection as a sedative to lessen the pain of childbirth. More blood tests and cultures were drawn to test for cancer and H.I.V. Thank GOD those came back negative as well. Every serious infectious disease test was coming out negative but the doctors were still scratching their heads because neither of them knew what my problem was.

It's already scary when you don't feel right medically but when even the doctors were drawing blanks it scared me half to death, literally. There were a few times when I broke down and cried. I couldn't help it. Doctors finally came up with the correct diagnosis: I had blood disorders from my immune system being confused. Due to all of the transplants I received, my immune system didn't recognize itself so it started producing antibodies against my white blood cells. In La-men's terms, it's known as auto-immune neutropenia.

Each time you receive a transplanted organ, your body has to adapt to it and my body has had to adapt to three livers on three separate occasions in my life. They first thought that my bone marrow was causing the problem and that it wasn't releasing white blood cells into my bloodstream like it should've been doing. For them to investigate this, I had to undergo a bone marrow biopsy. This particular biopsy was by far, the most painful procedure I've ever had to endure without anesthesia. Although I was sedated, <u>never</u> have I ever felt such excruciating pain than on that day.

It turned out that my bone marrow was performing normally but that my white blood cells were being destroyed through my splene (which filters the blood of any toxins and germs). My doctors then thought that with other methods and minor procedures, my problem would cure itself and that a splenectomy would be the absolute last resort if all else failed. I was prescribed numerous different medicines and more I.V. fluids to help combat my white blood cell deficiency.

I had to take so many pills including methadones for pain that I had lost my appetite for a couple weeks and I unfortunately lost between 10 to 15 pounds. I was already a small-framed young man and I've always been that way since birth because of my metabolism but all of those pills put such a thick thrush coat on my tongue that I couldn't taste anything. Seriously, I couldn't taste anything, not even sweets. It was enough to make me slip into another bout of depression. I might be skinny but I love to eat just as much the obese.

All other methods failed and the invasive splenectomy was carried out. Just four hours had passed since I was wheeled back into my hospital room from my surgery when who should walk in my room again? None other than those damn physical therapists! Understand, they are under precise orders from the doctors to help patients move around to help the blood circulate through the body better and help prevent clots but empathize from the patient's perspective though. I really don't feel like moving around right after a major surgery because I don't have the strength to move and I'm also still hurting. Hello?!

The whole three month hospital stay was extremely exhausting and I was discharged to go home for good on July 19, 2005 but I still had some difficulty maintaining my energy level from being blood cell deficient for so long. I stayed on a steady number of scheduled outpatient neupogen injections to boost up my white count. Can you believe for the hundredth time that I incidentally became jaundiced from my liver again? Luckily, this time the problem was steadily remedied with an enlarged dosage of my immuno-suppressive medication called prograf but it was not a quick fix.

Having to deal with a serious illness like this over and over again is mind-boggling because if you don't pre-occupy your mind and your time with other thoughts and activities then you'll literally go mentally insane. All kinds of negative thought will cloud your head while you're jaundiced and it's incredibly easy to start feeling sorry for yourself when you notice your appearance changing right in front of your eyes.

CHAPTER 7
My Unsuspecting Hobby

A turning point in my life occurred in November of 2004. It was after the break-up of my ex and I and just before my last hospital stay. I picked up the hobby of writing poetry and spoken-word. It originally started as an idea of mine to create the best personal profile for myself on a dateline. To my surprise, I received numerous responses from women. I re-developed a self-esteem problem when my ex and I stopped seeing each other romantically and I wanted to see if I still had that "something special" about myself that would intrigue a woman.

I continued to change my profile five times a month just to see how creative I could be. I met a lot of people off the line and made some friends as well. It's very encouraging to receive some positive feedback from time to time. Writing started out as just an innocent bobby at first but I began writing so much that it slowly became one of my passions. I carried my poetry book around with me everywhere I went, even while I was in my hospital bed anticipating that splenectomy procedure. Interestingly enough, the more I wrote, the more my inner self began to evolve. I then started to begin to get more comfortable with sharing my thought with other people, especially with women. I noticed this sense of change and enlightenment coming over me.

Suddenly, I started coming out of my shell and comfort zone of being so shy for so long. I used to fear what other people thought of me but nowadays, I don't care. Nobody knows me better than me. Nobody takes care of me but me. At the end of the day, I have to sleep with myself and I have to look myself in the mirror every morning. My love for writing led me to venture out to dinner theatres around town that had "open mic" nights and I actually got onstage on a few occasions. I still currently write in my poetry book at least three times a week before I go to sleep at night. I write poems among other things in my book including lyrics and short stories.

CHAPTER 8
It's Not Over for Me...

I just recently enrolled back in school this past May of 2006. A major in "Communications" interested me so I took a speech course. I originally made my first attempt to go to college back in the fall of 1999 right after I graduated from High School but I took a bunch of prerequisite courses that didn't really add up to any <u>real</u> college credits (don't even stress me on all the money I wasted). Then I took a few culinary courses because I used to swear up and down that I wanted to be a chef but after taking only four classes, I had had enough of my classes and came to the realization that I didn't want to be a damn chef. That wasn't where my heart was at anyway so I quit school completely in 2001 to start working full-time.

From 2001 to 2006, I managed to quit school, meet my daughter's mother, have a baby, get evicted from two apartments and lose three jobs only to come right back home and start the whole learning process all over again. I had to go back to school to make a better way of life for myself. I know I have to be able to provide for my daughter but even if she wasn't here, I would still need to make a better quality of living for myself. Daddy might <u>look</u> strong but daddy needs help.

Besides, unskilled labor seemed to be the only line of work I was perpetually stuck in. I always had to take the jobs that paid low wages, had huge turnover and virtually had <u>no</u> job security whatsoever. Getting in trouble became way too easy for me to accomplish. All I had to do to get written-up or fired was either wink an eye at a female co-worker or accidentally fart in somebody's face. I'm using sarcasm here but do you see how unstable these types of jobs were and still are? So if you have kids or you know of a young one, please tell them to stay in school. It is not worth having to struggle for so long before you see any light at the end of the tunnel. There's nothing humble about being broke for the rest of your life.

Getting back to my latest re-enrollment in school this past Summer, I didn't know what my speech class had in store for me. At first before the class began, I was expecting my instructor to be an older more physically challenged looking woman but instead she looked good. Actually, she looked damn good.

Now, by this time, I felt as if my low self-esteem problem was non-existent and that I was virtually invulnerable to rejection. I went out on a limb and felt so invincible that I tried to hit on her. You know the right side of your brain that's responsible for your logical thinking and reasoning? Well, I pushed that side of my brain all the way to the back of my head for a moment. In fact, I just threw it the hell out of the window when I saw her. I mean, I've had an attractive teacher before but not like this one. I understood that I was there to learn but she was so beautiful to me that it amazing and downright distracting at the same time.

The naïve part of me was so infatuated that I personally dedicated a poem of interest and recited it on her business phone. Consequently, reality attacked me with a vengeance the next class day when she confronted me about it. Basically she was very flattered by my words but said that our relationship had to be kept strictly professional (instructor to student). I'd be lying if I said that at that point I didn't feel awkward but on this specific occasion, I quickly saved face.

My confidence popped right back into place and my internal dialogue started telling me to continue to pursue her and hopefully she'll start to succumb but fortunately for my sake, I paid her enough respect to keep my head in my book though. I gradually got through the class, did everything I had to do and left when the term was over like everybody else did. I really do hope that our paths will cross again, perhaps in a different setting the next time but even if it doesn't happen, it's not the end of the world.

CHAPTER 9
My Aspirations

To wrap things up, I'm kind of glad everything that has transpired has already taken place. Who was better cut out to handle all that I have endured? God bless my hard-working grandfather for giving me such an unfathomable nickname. I'm not trying to toot my own horn here but it fits me like nothing else. Rock perseveres through hardships and stays solid even when everything else is collapsing around it.

There is still a little kid inside of me who isn't afraid to have fun and knows the value of a genuinely warm smile. I love to laugh and make other people laugh. Life is short and you never know just how stressful and heart-breaking it can be until your back is up against the wall and you're caught between a rock and a hard place (get it. rock?). If all that has happened to me never would've happened at all, I wouldn't have had the insight to write at all. I would still be a very lost individual emotionally trying to "find myself". I try to be the best person I can be on a daily basis but it's an ongoing battle as with the struggle of being human.

Lastly, if all goes well with my writing, I plan to work with it until I'm on my deathbed. My dream is to be a writer of original dramas for cable networks like "HBO" and "Showtime". I have something to say and I will not stop just because a few people choose to think otherwise. My writing is mostly adult oriented and usually meant for mature audiences but I've also written some wholesome manuscripts. I'm aiming more towards the "grown and sexy" who need to hear something different from just the same, the average and the mundane. I'm young, black, spontaneous, eager and very willing. Somewhere out there, there's somebody who knows exactly what I'm saying and those are the people I'm trying to reach out and touch.

Now that I'm 27 years young, I <u>will</u> place myself on the map before I die. I'm going to make my family and my daughter proud of me. Most importantly of all, I'm going to make myself proud of me. I really want to thank all of whom are reading my story for letting me take you on my virtuous journey of personal excellence. There's a small part of me that still is shy but once I warm up to the person I'm around then I'm good. I appreciate your time, thank you.

LaVergne, TN USA
08 April 2011
223475LV00002B/57/A